## THE DRUGLESS "DRUGS"

Depression, migraine, insomnia, lethargy — all are conventionally treated with drugs which are not always effective, often are addictive and have other menacing side effects. Yet these conditions, and others, have yielded to treatment with the vital amino acids, natural to the human system rather than being alien inorganic substances. Memory has been sharpened and aging retarded by programs of amino-acid supplementation.

For maintenance or restoration of good health, the proper balance of amino acids in the body is a necessity. This concise guide gives the facts about amino acids and how you can use them for enhanced and enduring well-being.

## ABOUT THE AUTHOR AND EDITORS

**Robert Garrison, Jr., R.Ph., M.A.,** received his Pharmacy degree from the University of Washington and his Master's degree in Adult Education and Training from San Diego State University. In addition to his extensive experience in pharmacy management, Mr. Garrison has spent over ten years as a nutritional consultant to physicians, psychologists, corporations and county substance abuse programs. He is an instructor in pharmacology and nutrition for San Diego Community College and Executive Director of the California Institute for Contemporary Education. He has just completed a soon to be published study on subclinical malnutrition and learning behavior among high school students. Among the many national organizations for health enhancement to which Mr. Garrison belongs are the Pharmacists' Society for Nutrition Education, the San Diego County Advisory Committee on Drug Abuse and the Society for Nutrition Education.

**Richard A. Passwater, Ph.D.,** is one of the most called-upon authorities for information relating to preventive health care. A noted biochemist, he is credited with popularizing the term "super-nutrition" largely as a result of having written two bestsellers on the subject: *Supernutrition – Megavitamin Revolution* and *Supernutrition for Healthy Hearts.* His other books include *Easy No-Flab Diet, Cancer and Its Nutritional Therapies,* and the recently published *Selenium as Food & Medicine.* He has just completed a new book on *Hair Analysis* with Elmer M. Cranton, M.D.

**Earl Mindell, R.Ph., Ph.D.,** combines the expertise and working experience of a pharmacist with extensive knowledge in most of the nutrition areas. His book *Earl Mindell's Vitamin Bible* is now a million-copy bestseller; and his more recent *Vitamin Bible for Your Kids* may very well duplicate his first *Bible's* publishing history. Dr. Mindell's popular *Quick & Easy Guide to Better Health* was just published by Keats Publishing.

# LYSINE, TRYPTOPHAN AND OTHER AMINO ACIDS

## FOOD FOR OUR BRAINS …
## MAINTENANCE FOR OUR BODIES

by Robert Garrison, Jr., R.Ph., M.A.

Keats Publishing, Inc. New Canaan, Connecticut

*Lysine, Tryptophan and Other Amino Acids* is not intended as medical advice. Its intention is solely informational and educational. Please consult a medical or health professional should the need for one be warranted.

# Contents

# I AMINO ACIDS AND THE MAKING OF PROTEINS

Natural sleep aid, antidepressant, baldness cure, anti-aging supplement, appetite suppressant, stimulant, smart pill, herpes cure, are just a few of the claims being made today for amino acid supplements. But most of the contemporary claims for beneficial effects of amino acids as individual supplements are unrelated to the traditional role attributed to amino acids in most nutrition books. You've probably read somewhere along the way that amino acids have something to do with protein. Indeed, they are the component parts of protein. And before we look at the individual amino acids, it may be helpful to look first at the diversity of functions amino acids play when they work together as proteins. Then we will look at some potential uses of individual amino acids as therapeutic agents.

Protein is basic to a sound nutritional program and good health. Many people think of protein as being synonymous with steak and sound nutrition, an assumption which is not very accurate. Some of the roles played by protein include the building of body tissues, the repairing of body tissues and the maintenance of body tissues. All of these functions are exclusive roles played by protein, although other nutrients can play supporting roles.

But protein is also necessary to make bone, to form blood cells and to make antibodies, the substances the body uses to fight infection. And the chemical and physical reactions inside each cell that constitute the very life of that cell, and therefore the life of the whole body are all regulated by proteins called enzymes.

If the proteins which act as enzymes are altered, the detrimental effects will be seen in every situation where that protein was to assist a given reaction. For example, let's say that an unstable chemical such as a peroxide reacts with another substance in the body which in turn reacts with DNA and RNA (protein-like substances which form a vital part of the nucleus of every cell in the body). DNA and RNA work together to tell which amino acids go where to create a protein molecule. If the function of DNA and RNA is impaired, the protein is constructed incorrectly. If the body's immunological defense system no longer recognizes these incorrectly constructed proteins, it attacks them as it would any foreign proteins, bacteria or viruses. Then the body becomes its own enemy. And likewise, if the enzymes consisting of protein are constructed incorrectly, their necessary biochemical functions do not get performed and an endless number of malfunctions can ensue. Distorted DNA and RNA and the resulting protein mis-synthesis are now believed to play a significant role in the aging process.[1,2]

Not only are proteins dependent upon DNA and RNA to transfer the genetic coding for proper construction, but certain amino acids are required for the repair of the DNA and RNA should they become damaged. We will take a closer look at some of these amino acids and their potential in slowing down the aging process in the next section.

Proteins not functioning as enzymes might take on the role of hormones, substances which are manufactured within cells in one part of the body, then leave the area, toddle around in the body fluids and finally exert their influence on cells in another area.

Proteins can play additional roles. They can act as oxygen carriers, they can participate in muscular contraction, and they can have relationships with genes. Proteins are exceptionally talented indeed!

What are the characteristics of proteins that make them so talented and capable of playing so many roles? The answer to this question can be found by looking at the structure of protein.

The manner in which the amino acids are put together to form a given protein determines how and where that protein will exert its influence. Amino acids are the components of protein and protein is the sum of its amino acid parts.

The quality of the protein in the diet depends on the particular ratio of amino acids contained in that protein. The foods which contain protein with an amino acid ratio that closely resembles the amino acid of proteins in our bodies are said to be high quality protein. High quality protein foods are rated to have a high biological value. Foods with the highest biological value — meaning they have the best amino acid ratio for our bodies — include breast milk (which is given the top value of 100), whole-egg protein (94) and cow's milk (85). Meats, poultry and fish are rated between 86 and 76.

The idea that steak is synonymous with protein is not altogether correct. In addition to the fact that the steak may contain more fat than protein, high quality protein can also be found in vegetable foods. For example, rice has an amino acid ratio that allows it to be ranked with a biological value of 80. Potatoes have a high quality protein and are ranked with a biological value of 78. And vegetarians know that if a particular vegetable is low in one amino acid or another, by combining a different vegetable, grain or legume which is high in the missing amino acid, a meal with protein of high biological value can be obtained.

It is very important to understand that amino acids function together in a unique balance. An upset in this balance can lead to a variety of disorders. And these disorders are not only the direct result of a missing amino acid but can also be the indirect result of another amino acid becoming too concentrated. For example, gelatin is an imbalanced protein high in the amino acid glycine. If glycine levels become too high we produce excessive uric acid which can lead to gout.

Where the amino acids serve as precursors to other chemicals in the body, these chemicals may exist in a balanced relationship. Such is the case for the brain neurotransmitters serotonin, dopamine and norepinephrine. All three of these chemicals require certain amino acids for their synthesis. By altering the amount or ratio of the precursor amino acids, the balanced relationship between these neurotransmitters can be upset. This can lead to behavioral disorders on the one hand, or can be the basis for the therapeutic use of certain amino acids on the other.

Some amino acids are "essential" or indispensable dietary constituents because our bodies cannot manufacture them. Other amino acids are categorized as "nonessential" or dispensable since they can be manufactured within the body. But this categorization is not entirely correct since many individuals cannot manufacture enough of the so-called "nonessential" amino acids and therefore it becomes essential that these individuals supplement their diet with those additional amino acids necessary to meet their needs.

The amino acids that are categorized as "essential" and must be obtained from the diet are histidine, isoleucine, leucine, lysine, methionine, phenylalanine, threonine, tryptophan and valine. There are two other amino acids that must be derived from these essential amino acids and probably should be classified as "essential." They are cysteine, which is made from methionine, and tyrosine, which is made from phenylalanine. Arginine is often listed as a nonessential amino acid but we really can't synthesize enough arginine to meet our needs and should include arginine as an essential amino acid.

In addition to these twelve amino acids which occur in proteins within the body cells, there are eight amino acids which are present in most proteins but may not be necessary in the diet since our bodies may be able to manufacture them from other sources. These include alanine, aspartic acid, asparagine, glutamic acid, glutamine, glycine, proline and serine. There are other related accessory food factors such as carnitine, which also may have important therapeutic uses.

Most of the amino acids can exist in two forms, one being the mirror image of the other. The form used to make protein has been designated as the L-series and therefore you may see an amino acid labeled as L-lysine. Many distributors of amino acid supplements simply drop the L and L-lysine then becomes just plain lysine.

The nature of any given protein is first determined by the sequence in which these amino acids are linked and the amounts of each amino acid present. The linkage between the amino acids is called a "peptide" link. When just two amino acids are linked they form what is called a "dipeptide." When three amino acids are linked they form what is called a "tripeptide" and so on. Proteins can consist of hundreds of these linkages.

Long chains of amino acids are called "polypeptide" chains and form proteins like that of muscle fibers, hair and collagen, an important constituent of connective tissue and bone which can be turned into gelatin by boiling. When the amino acids are linked together in a round or ellipsoidal manner they form proteins such as hemoglobin, insulin, albumins and globulins.

Two very short chain amino acid peptides called enkephalins act as natural painkillers in our body. They are very much like the opiate narcotic painkillers but they are manufactured in our own body and help the body handle great pain. These enkephalins are also involved in mood and the regulation of emotions. A larger amino acid chain that contains the short, five amino acid sequence of the enkephalins, is called beta-endorphin. It too has opiate activity like morphine and occurs naturally in the pituitary gland.

Amino acids are not acids in the sense that we normally think of acids. In fact most amino acids are neutral. But the chemical classification of amino acids as acids or bases is important to scientists in understanding how they get into the body and across membranes.

Enzymes in the gastric juice followed by enzymes from the pancreas and the small intestine·all work on the protein in the diet to break it down into its component dipeptides or individual amino acids. Once these amino acids are absorbed they are transported to the liver for distribution throughout the body as needed.

Over the last few years there has been a great deal of excitement over the use of individual amino acid supplements to treat everything from depression and baldness to aging. But two things should be kept in mind when considering supplementing with an individual amino acid:

**First:** Where amino acids act as precursors to other active agents in the body, they rarely act alone. Many other cofactors such as vitamins and minerals are often necessary to manufacture the final chemical from the particular amino acid. If any one of these cofactors is missing, increasing the amino acid availability by supplementing will not appreciably alter the synthesis or manufacturing process.

**Second:** Most amino acids compete with other amino acids. They compete for transportation into the body and at many other sites along the way to their final destination. So the therapeutic use of any single amino acid may be impaired by the presence of other amino acids. Excessive use of any single amino acid can therefore potentially inhibit the activity and availability of certain other amino acids. But as a pharmacist, let me assure you that the amino acids are far safer as therapeutic agents than most prescription drugs.

In the next section amino acids will be discussed as therapeutic agents. Due to the scope of this booklet, not all known functions of each amino acid will be presented.

# II AMINO ACIDS AS BRAIN FOODS AND OTHER THERAPEUTIC FUNCTIONS

In order to more fully understand the therapeutic applications of certain amino acids, we need to step inside our brains. In Michelangelo's painting, The Creation of Adam, God and Adam are reaching out to each other but their hands do not quite touch as God gives

Adam the divine spark, creating the soul of man. A similar event occurs in human brains.

Billions and billions of nerve cells in the brain reach out to each other and make perhaps as many as a quadrillion connections. At each connection a spark-like reaction takes place. When this happens, an electrical and a chemical impulse is transferred enabling us to think, to feel, to learn, to move, to remember and to sense the beautiful world around us.

These cells are called neurons and are like a microcomputer that processes information via thousands of connections. Each of these cells have similar structural components but no two cells are exactly alike. Extending from the cell body like branches from a tree are the dendrites. The dendrites act as receivers of signals from neighboring nerve cells.

There is one long fiber called the axon which extends from the cell body. At the end of the axon are more branches, and at their tips they have tiny little sacs. The axon is the transmitter which sends signals to other neurons.

When a neuron's dendrites receive an impulse from another neuron, a wave of electrical activity moves through the cell and if strong

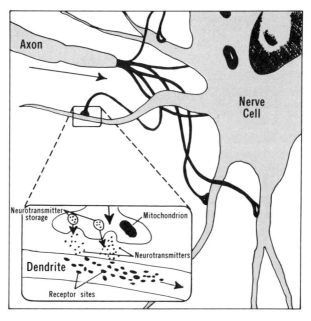

enough, will cause the cell to "fire." When the cell fires, the sac and the end of the axon bursts open and sends a chemical messenger called a neurotransmitter into the narrow space between the end of the axon and the next cell's dendrites. The neurotransmitter flows over to the receiving cell's dendrites, sparking a second electrical current. Once the chemical neurotransmitter has passed on its signal, it is either inactivated by enzymes or taken up and stored back in the sac at the end of the axon.

So what does all this have to do with amino acids? Some of the neurotransmitters are dependent on certain amino acids for their synthesis. By manipulating these amino acids through the use of amino acid supplements, the entire process described above can be altered, thereby potentially affecting mood, emotions, memory, arousal, sleep and many other related functions.

## PHENYLALANINE

**Source:** Phenylalanine occurs naturally in almost any good source of protein: beef, chicken, fish, eggs, soybeans, cottage cheese and milk. It also occurs in baked beans, peanuts and almonds.

**Function:** Phenylalanine is an amino acid which, among other functions, is used by the brain to manufacture norepinephrine. And among the many functions of norepinephrine, one function is as a neurotransmitter allowing certain brain cells to communicate with each other as described earlier. In this capacity, norepinephrine appears to play an important role in learning and memory.

When experimental animals are given drugs that are very specific for decreasing the amount of norepinephrine in the brain, scientists find that the animal's capacity for learning is blocked. And when the animals are then given an injection of norepinephrine their learning capacity returns.

Normally, when norepinephrine is not helping brain cells communicate with each other, it is stored in little tiny pouches at the end of neurons located in the brain. When it becomes necessary for norepinephrine to transmit impulses to another cell, it is released from these pouches, "talks" to another cell and then is returned to its pouch.

Drugs such as amphetamines and Ritalin block norepinephrine from reentering these pouches and thereby increase the amount of norepinephrine transmitting messages. These types of drugs seem to promote memory and improve learning by increasing the attentiveness of the learner and the learner's ability to focus. But once the nerves have released all their stored norepinephrine from the little pouches these stimulant drugs no longer have any affect on learning behavior. And when this tolerance takes place the decreased stimulation is often accompanied by depression.

Norepinephrine requires a number of nutrients for its synthesis: pterin, oxygen, iron, vitamin B6, vitamin C, the mineral copper and the amino acid tyrosine. Tyrosine is derived from the amino acid phenylalanine. Since phenylalanine is the raw material from which norepinephrine is manufactured, it has been suggested that perhaps a phenylalanine supplement might improve learning and might be useful in the treatment of some types of depression. Certain types of depression have responded very favorably to phenylalanine and there have been reports suggesting attention span and therefore learning may be improved with this amino acid. (See the tyrosine section for a discussion of its potential as an antidepressant.)

As mentioned in the previous chapter, when neurotransmitters such as norepinephrine have completed their mission they are either inactivated by enzymes or restored in the sacs at the ends of the axons. In the case of norepinephrine, the enzyme monoamine oxidase (MAO) is responsible for inactivating this neurotransmitter. Sometime around the age of forty-five the levels of MAO increase to a point where greater than normal amounts of norepinephrine are necessary to initiate transmission. Therefore, the older we get the more important it becomes to provide all the necessary ingredients for the synthesis of norepinephrine, including the amino acid phenylalanine.

Some have suggested that phenylalanine may be an effective appetite suppressant and diet aid. Theoretically, this amino acid should help control appetite while one is trying to change overall eating habits. Decreasing fat intake and sugars while increasing the consumption of wholegrain bread and fresh vegetables, and supplementing with phenylalanine during the transition period may be the answer to that long sought after weight maintenance program. If you have high blood pressure and are trying to lose weight with the aid of phenylalanine, don't forget to monitor your blood pressure during this period.

You might be interested in this additional note on phenylalanine. Soon a new synthetic sweetener will adorn soft drinks from coast to coast in an attempt to perfect our nation's number one beverage. When phenylalanine is combined with the amino acid known as aspartic acid, it forms this new sweetener aspartame.

# TRYPTOPHAN

**Source:** Tryptophan is present in high quality protein foods such as fish, chicken, eggs, beef, soybeans and milk. Tryptophan is present in only very small amounts in the legumes. Therefore, in order to improve the quality of protein available from legumes, foods high in tryptophan, such as the grains, seeds and nuts should be added to the meal. Corn based diets are usually deficient in this amino acid.

**Function:**

*TRYPTOPHAN AND NIACIN INTERRELATIONSHIP:* As early as 1913 it was noted that the disease pellagra was due to a deficiency of tryptophan in maize. But confusion set in when additional research demonstrated that a non-amino acid substance in yeast could prevent pellagra. It took another thirty years before it was determined that the vitamin nicotinic acid or niacin was actually the anti-pellagra vitamin and that the body could manufacture niacin from dietary tryptophan if the diet was inadequate in niacin. Therefore, tryptophan serves an important function in assuring the body of adequate amounts of niacin.

In order for tryptophan to be metabolized properly it requires vitamin B6. When there is inadequate B6 present a derangement of tryptophan metabolism occurs and a substance called xanthurenic acid is excreted in the urine. This property of tryptophan metabolism makes this amino acid a fairly good test for vitamin B6 adequacy and when utilized in this manner it is called the tryptophan load test. And because tryptophan uses vitamin B6 in the body, it may be necessary to increase vitamin B6 intake when supplementing the diet with tryptophan.

TRYPTOPHAN AND BRAIN FUNCTION: Much of the recent excitement centering around this amino acid supplement is due to its relationship with the neurotransmitter in the brain called serotonin. Serotonin was first isolated from intestinal cells in 1937 by V. Erspamer. Serotonin is also found in other tissues bound with various substances, such as histamine and heparin. In 1947 I.H. Page showed it to be a substance involved in the clotting of blood and in 1953 he demonstrated serotonin's presence in the brain.

Serotonin is found in blood platelets in a bound state. During the clotting process, serotonin is released and helps prevent bleeding by constricting blood vessels around the injury.[3] Excessive bleeding during a full moon or ion wind is apparently caused by the release of the anticoagulant heparin from the serotonin complexes.

Serotonin occurs naturally in vegetables as well as in animals. There are large amounts of it in unripe bananas. Matoke is a species of banana that is eaten green and is consumed in large quantities by many Africans. This heavy consumption raises serotonin levels considerably and can result in cardiovascular disorders.[4,5]

Serotonin requires a number of compounds for its synthesis in our bodies — pterin, oxygen, iron, vitamin B6 as well as tryptophan. Since the early 1960s researchers have been debating the usefulness of tryptophan supplements to manipulate serotonin levels selectively in the treatment of depression and sleep disorders.

TRYPTOPHAN FOR DEPRESSION: Affective disorders, mania and depression, are characterized by changes in mood state as the primary symptoms. These mood extremes can be accompanied by delusions and disordered thought. The use of tryptophan in these disorders has been approached in two different ways: 1. The biochemical approach where attempts are made to correlate mood with levels of tryptophan and serotonin in various tissues; and 2. The clinical approach where the subject is given tryptophan and the antidepressant effects are measured under formal research conditions. A look at the research that has gone on in both of these approaches is useful in determining whether tryptophan supplements should be used to replace some more expensive and potentially dangerous prescription drugs.

In 1973 a research study correlated free plasma tryptophan levels with plasma estrogen levels in postmenopausal women with depression.[6] Then these women were given estrogen and mood was improved along with an increase in plasma-free tryptophan.

Emotional instability and depression are common occurrences in women who have just given birth. A 1976 study correlated mood and tryptophan levels in eighteen women during the postpartum period. The women who had clinical signs of severe depression had free plasma tryptophan levels similar to those found in depressive illnesses.[7]

Additional research back in 1965 and 1946 also showed a relationship between mood and free tryptophan levels in the plasma.[8,9] Bridges' research in 1976 suggests that there may be a specific group of individuals suffering from depression who might respond favorably to tryptophan, possibly combined with the amino acid tyrosine.[10]

In another major study carried out in Scandinavia, tryptophan was compared with the drug imipramine, a popular antidepressant often prescribed under the brand name Tofranil. The findings from this study showed tryptophan to be just as effective as imipramine. And since tryptophan is a natural amino acid, the side effects with the tryptophan group were much less frequent and less severe than the group treated with imipramine.[11] In 1975 and in 1978 similar findings were reported.[12,13]

The drug amitriptyline, which is sold under the brand names of Elavil and Endep, was compared to the effectiveness of tryptophan in alleviating depression by Herrington in 1976.[14] Both groups improved at the same rate and there appeared to be no differences between the group treated with the amitriptyline and the group treated with the amino acid tryptophan. But the tryptophan-treated group held up much better over a six month follow-up period! The drug-treated group had a greater tendency to relapse.

So what is the bottom line regarding tryptophan as an antidepressant? It appears that this natural amino acid has antidepressant action comparable to that of the commonly prescribed drugs, imipramine and amitriptyline.

*TRYPTOPHAN FOR SLEEP:* It has been fairly well established that the neurotransmitter serotonin plays a major role in inducing sleep. Therefore it seems logical that tryptophan should be tested as a natural aid to sleep since, as we have discussed, tryptophan is the precursor to serotonin.

And indeed, research has taken place for over fifteen years to determine if tryptophan could possibly replace some of the drugs used for sleep which can be habit forming. Cooper summarized this research in 1979 and concluded that tryptophan as a sleep aid significantly decreased the time necessary to fall asleep. He concluded that it also significantly increased the duration of sleep and perhaps improved the quality of sleep.[15]

One of the major advantages of tryptophan as a replacement for sleeping pills is that it doesn't interfere with the ability to drive an automobile the next day. But there are two criteria that must be followed to use tryptophan as an effective sleep aid. First, the tryptophan supplement must be taken at night. Apparently, there is an enzyme that prevents the necessary concentration of tryptophan to induce sleep. This enzyme is quite active during the day but takes a break at night.

Second: It is necessary to remove any competitive amino acids from the area known as the "blood brain barrier." The tryptophan must pass this barrier and can do so much more readily if there are no other amino acids trying to get through at the same time. This can be accomplished by eating a complex carbohydrate meal with little or no protein as the last meal of the day. Then take the tryptophan supplement and little competition to get into the brain will exist.

*TRYPTOPHAN FOR MIGRAINE:* John A. Brainard, M.D., in his book *Control of Migraine,* lists the following as primary offenders that can trigger a migraine headache in sensitive individuals: alcohol, monosodium glutamate (that flavor enhancer added to unpalatable food and frequently used in Chinese restaurants), nitroglycerine (a prescription drug for angina), and a sudden increase in salt intake.[16]

Dr. Federigo Sicuteri studied serotonin levels in migraine patients and found that they had a lower than normal level of this neurotransmitter. And since, as we have already seen, tryptophan is the precursor for serotonin synthesis, Dr. Sicuteri reasoned that tryptophan supplements may be effective in treating migraine sufferers. He found this amino acid to be effective in about half of the migraine sufferers treated.[17]

Dr. Sicuteri's findings are consistent with other research that showed a drop in blood serotonin levels during a migraine attack.[18] These studies also showed that there was an increase in the level of free fatty acids. This is interesting because some reports from migraine sufferers relate their attack with fasting or the beginning of a weight-loss diet. During these situations the free fatty acids in the blood are elevated. They are also elevated during emotional stress and with alcohol consumption, both of which have been implicated as migraine triggers. These free fatty acids may somehow be responsible for the low serotonin levels during a migraine attack.

TRYPTOPHAN FOR IMMUNITY: Antibodies roam around in the blood defending the body against foreign substances. They are a major line of defense to protect us from disease. And they give rise to the allergy response when we become sensitized to certain foods or substances in our environment.

These antibodies are made by a special type of white blood cell called B-lymphocytes (B stands for bone marrow, where they originate). In animal studies, a deficiency of the amino acid tryptophan has been shown to inhibit the antibody-forming response. Similar nutrients whose deficiency can impair this response include: pyridoxine, folic acid, pantothenic acid, thiamine, riboflavin, niacin, protein, vitamin A and vitamin C.[19]

Tryptophan can be an exciting therapeutic agent. For short term usage it certainly is much safer than its prescription drug counterparts. More information is needed to evaluate its effects when used in high doses for long term therapy.

# GLUTAMINE (GLUTAMIC ACID)

**Source:** Glutamic acid is the most prominent amino acid in wheat protein.

**Function:** Glutamine is the amide form of glutamic acid, a "non-essential" amino acid that may improve intelligence, speed the healing of ulcers and give a "lift" from fatigue. It may also help control alcoholism, certain types of schizophrenia and the craving for sweets. Dosages between 1 and 4 grams (1,000 to 4,000 milligrams) daily have been prescribed.

Dr. Roger Williams and associates at the Clayton Foundation for Research, University of Texas have carried out extensive research on L-glutamine. Their studies have shown that glutamine consistently decreases the craving for alcohol consumption in the alcoholic patient. It should be noted that glutamic acid does not work as well as glutamine and should not be used in place of glutamine.[20]


# III THE SULFUR-CONTAINING AMINO ACIDS


The sulfur-containing amino acids are methionine, cysteine, cystine and taurine. They are placed in a separate section here because sulfur is such an important essential nutrient. Sulfur in its dietary form is a powerful aid in protecting against radiation and pollution. And in addition, it plays a role in slowing down the aging process and extending lifespan. The sulfur-containing amino acids function as antioxidants, free-radical deactivators, neutralizers of toxins, and as aids to protein synthesis.

An average adult body contains about 140 grams of sulfur. Approximately 850 mg of sulfur is lost every day and must be replaced. The best source of sulfur is in the form of sulfur amino acids, and the best source of sulfur amino acids is eggs. Since humans cannot use elemental sulfur to make the sulfur amino acids, we must get our sulfur in the diet. One egg supplies approximately 65 mg of sulfur and one gram of the amino acid cysteine, which as cysteine hydrochloride supplies approximately 180 mg of sulfur.[21]

Vitamin C, to a certain extent, is converted in the body to a form that requires sulfur. Those who are supplementing with large doses of vitamin C may be placing demands on their sulfur reserves and may need extra amounts of the sulfur-containing amino acids.

The sulfur amino acids serve a useful role as natural carriers of the trace element selenium. In this role they facilitate the action of selenium as a potent protector against cancer and a major compound for slowing down the aging process.

# METHIONINE

**Source:** Methionine is abundant in chicken, beef, fish, ham, eggs, cottage cheese, liver, sardines and milk. Many vegetables and legumes are weak in methionine and therefore must be combined with grains, seeds or nuts (not peanuts) to improve the overall protein quality.

**Function:** Methionine is a member of the lipotropic team which includes choline, inositol and betaine. Its primary function, as a lipotropic, is to prevent excessive accumulation of fat in the liver. By increasing the liver's production of lecithin, methionine helps prevent cholesterol buildup.

As mentioned earlier, methionine also serves an important role in providing the trace element sulfur. The other amino acids that also provide us with sulfur, cysteine, cystine and taurine, can be made in the body as long as we consume adequate amounts of the essential amino acid methionine. But this can put a tremendous burden on our methionine supply. If we consume a diet that is deficient in the amino acid cysteine, our methionine requirements will go up approximately 30 percent.

Every body cell contains sulfur, with the greatest concentration in the cells of skin, hair and joints. Keratin, the horny layer of skin, has a high concentration of sulfur and so do fingernails, toenails and hair. In fact, curly hair is due to the sulfur bonding in the hair — when curly hair is straightened, these sulfur bonds are rearranged. So methionine is very important as the principal supplier of sulfur, to prevent disorders of the skin and nails.

Methionine and the other sulfur-containing amino acids also play an important role as antioxidants, free-radical deactivators and neutralizers of certain toxins. All of these activities help to slow down the aging process.

A property of these sulfur amino acids that helps eliminate those highly reactive chemicals known as free-radicals is their ability to chelate or grab onto certain metallic cations such as copper. This ability to chelate heavy metals helps to eliminate the build-up of toxic minerals such as lead, mercury and cadmium.

Since methionine falls into the category known as "methyl donors," it has been included in nutritional supplement formulas as an anti-fatigue agent.

## TAURINE

One of the amino acids that can be made from methionine is taurine. Taurine helps stabilize the excitability of membranes which is very important in the control of epileptic seizures. Research is currently underway to determine if taurine may be a better approach to epilepsy than such drugs such as Dilantin and phenobarbital. Taurine and sulfur may be factors necessary for the control of many disorders, including some of the biochemical changes that take place in the aging process.

One factor that may contribute to an increased need for methionine and its derivatives is its loss of activity with excessive alcohol consumption. One of the breakdown products of methionine has been found at high plasma levels in alcoholics suggesting that too much alcohol may destroy methionine.[23]

Methionine is also used by the body to make choline, another brain food which plays an important role in memory. One way to conserve methionine is to provide a dietary source of choline so that methionine is not needed for choline synthesis. The best source of natural choline is lecithin. Therefore, supplementing your diet with lecithin, among other things, helps to conserve the important sulfur amino acid, methionine.

One particular disease state where methionine intake must be restricted is homocystinuria. These individuals can't metabolize methionine properly and must supplement their low methionine diet with the amino acid cystine.

# CYSTEINE AND CYSTINE

**Source:** Available primarily from eggs, milk, beef and wheat.

**Function:** The amino acid cysteine is very unstable and is readily converted to the amino acid cystine. Since most cysteine supplements have probably undergone conversion to cystine, we will discuss the properties of these two amino acids by referring just to cystine.

The important roles cystine plays have been discussed under the general heading of the sulfur containing amino acids. These include its function as an antioxidant and free-radical deactivator, a detoxifying agent, an immune system improver and a DNA repair aid. In these roles cystine plays a powerful role in protecting against pollution and radiation and probably extending lifespan.

As an antioxidant, cystine works closely with vitamin E and selenium. Each of these nutrients enhance the antioxidant role of the other.

Dr. Eustace Barton-Wright of London's Greenwich and District Hospitals has been using nutritional supplements in the treatment of arthritis, both osteoarthritis and rheumatoid. The technique of using 100 mg of pantothenic acid produced favorable results only when the amino acid cystine was added to the regimen.[22]

Recently, Dr. William Philpott has suggested that cystine is necessary for the utilization of vitamin B6. Dr. Philpott explains that "a majority of chronic degenerative illnesses, whether physical or mental, have a vitamin B6 utilization disorder. The culprit in this vitamin

B6 utilization problem seems to be L-cystine deficiency." He recommends that patients who have the vitamin B6 utilization problem take 1.5 grams of L-cystine three times a day for a month and then reduce the amount to twice daily.[24]

# IV ACCESSORY AMINO ACIDS

## TYROSINE

**Source:** Aged cheese, beer, wine, yeast, ripe bananas, avocado, pickled herring and chicken livers.

**Function:** Tyrosine is another amino acid that is in that grey zone between being classified as an essential or nonessential amino acid. If the diet is deficient in this amino acid, the requirement for phenylalanine goes up since tyrosine can be synthesized from phenylalanine. If an individual has difficulty in converting phenylalanine to tyrosine, or wants to conserve phenylalanine for other duties, dietary tyrosine must be included.

This amino acid plays an intermediary role in the synthesis of the neurotransmitter norepinephrine from the amino acid phenylalanine. The potential use of phenylalanine as a dietary supplement in this capacity has already been discussed.

Just as phenylalanine is being investigated as a useful agent in treating mental disorders, so too is the amino acid tyrosine. Dr. Alan J. Gelenberg of the Department of Psychiatry of Harvard Medical School has found that tyrosine plays a role in controlling anxiety and depression. He suggests that a lack of available tyrosine results in a deficiency of the neurotransmitter norepinephrine at a specific site in the brain, which in turn, relates to mood problems such as depression. Dr. Gelenberg reported considerable improvement in two patients whose longstanding depressions were not responsive to conventional drug therapy. At a dosage of 100 mg of tyrosine daily for two weeks, one patient was able to discontinue the drug amphetamine and the other was able to reduce the amphetamine intake to a minimal level.[25]

Tyrosine has been mentioned earlier as a potential trigger of migraine headaches. This may be due to its breakdown product called tyramine. Tyrosine breaks down to tyramine in such foods as aged cheese, beer, wine, yeast, ripe bananas, avocado, pickled herring and chicken livers. Eliminating these foods from the diet of sensitive individuals may be an effective way to eliminate migraine headaches.

This breakdown product tyramine, when ingested in combination with the antidepressants of the class known as monoamine oxidase inhibitors (MAOI), can cause a serious increase in blood pressure. This is why the above mentioned foods are eliminated when a patient is prescribed a MAOI drug. It certainly seems as though amino acid supplements are much safer than drugs in the treatment of depression.

One additional note on tyrosine; it has been suggested that tyrosine in combination with tryptophan may be a better sleep aid than tryptophan alone.[10]

# LEUCINE, ISOLEUCINE AND VALINE

**Source:** These three amino acids are adequately supplied in the diet, at least for most individuals, from any good protein source including chicken, fish, beef, soybeans, eggs, cottage cheese, liver, baked beans and milk. Certain grains, seeds and nuts, and most vegetables do not have adequate amounts of isoleucine and therefore need to be complemented in the diet with legumes.

**Function:** Leucine, isoleucine and valine cannot be manufactured by the body and must be supplied in the diet. They follow similar metabolic pathways providing ingredients for the manufacturing of other essential biochemical components in the body, some of which are utilized for the production of energy.

**Related disorders:** The three amino acids are normally metabolized through a series of steps into simple acids. But in the disease known as "maple syrup urine" these amino acids are not completely broken down and end up in the urine. The urine has an odor of maple syrup and is a valuable clue in the diagnosis of this disease.

Infants with maple syrup urine disease appear normal at birth but within a few days are unable to suck or swallow properly. They may have seizures and if they survive, mental retardation is severe. Restrictive diets have helped but the infant will not have weight gain without some supply of these three amino acids.

Another inborn error of metabolism that just involves the amino acid leucine is leucine-induced hypoglycemia. At about the fourth month of life the infant with this disease may begin to have convulsions, slowed growth, delayed mental development and symptoms much like Cushing's syndrome, including obesity, acne, osteoporosis and facial hair growth. Since all protein foods contain leucine, it is impossible to treat these infants with a diet that has the leucine removed without removing all protein from the diet. But by careful manipulation of the diet the child may be able to tolerate a normal diet by the age of five or six years when the disease has run its course.

# LYSINE

**Source:** Lysine is found in all high quality proteins such as fish, chicken, egg and milk but is deficient in the grains, seeds and nuts. Therefore, to maximize the available protein from grains, seeds and nuts they should be combined with eggs, milk or garbanzo beans.

Strict vegetarians may require supplementation with lysine.

**Function:** One very important function of lysine is to assure adequate absorption of the mineral calcium. Another function of this amino acid is in the formation of collagen. Collagen is a widely distributed protein that makes up the matrix of bone, cartilage and connective tissue. Before lysine can be utilized in the formation of collagen, it must be converted to another form. This conversion process is regulated by vitamin C. So here we see an example of the fascinating interrelationship of the various nutrients. Without vitamin C or adequate protein to supply the amino acid lysine, our wounds would not heal properly and we would become more susceptible to infection.

Lysine can enter metabolic pathways that eventually provide necessary ingredients for the production of energy. This is true of many of the amino acids and is the reason protein can be a source of energy or calories. But ordinarily the body reserves protein and its amino acid components for the maintenance and repair of tissue rather than converting the amino acids into energy.

One relatively new use for lysine is in the symptomatic treatment of herpes simplex. This viral infection is more commonly known as cold sores or fever blisters. Herpes has become a major venereal disease in the United States and can cause serious complications in babies who contract the disease from the mother during birth.

In order to fully appreciate the potential of lysine in controlling the painful and stubborn blisters brought on by the herpes infection, let's look at the work of Doctors Chris Kagan and R.W. Tankersley. Dr. Kagan, while working in the viral lab at the Cedars of Lebanon Hospital in Los Angeles (he is currently with the Permanente Medical Group in Oakland, CA), noted that the amino acid arginine was always added to the solution used to grow tissue cells infected with the herpes virus. Dr. Tankersley at the University of Richmond had previously determined that in order for the herpes virus to grow, arginine must be added to the solution. And that when lysine was added to the growth media, the virus did not grow.[26]

It was Dr. Kagan then who suggested that if arginine favored the virus and lysine inhibited it, why not use lysine clinically as a therapy for herpes infection?[27] So Dr. Kagan, Dr. Richard S. Griffith, Professor of Medicine at the Indiana University School of Medicine, and Dr. Arthur L. Norins, Professor of Dermatology at the same medical school, all got together to try this new approach.

These researchers found lysine suppressed symptoms of herpes in 96 percent of the forty-five patients tested. Several patients were studied for as long as three years, with complete remission of the herpes and no adverse reactions observed. Their report stated: "The pain disappeared abruptly overnight in virtually every instance, new vesicles (blisters) failed to appear, and resolution in the majority was considered to be more rapid than in their past experience. The initiating lesion remained confined to one area in those patients who characteristically had experienced extension and progression to multiple sites. Patients had rapid control of their initial lesion and obtained continued suppression while on lysine. Patients were infection-free while on lysine but found within one to four weeks after stopping lysine, return of the lesions could be predicted."[28]

Inactive herpes can be controlled in most individuals with just one 500 milligram tablet or capsule of L-lysine daily. But sometimes a larger dose is necessary for the first few months, such as one 500 milligram tablet three times daily for four to six months. There is more to be learned about herpes and its relationship with lysine and arginine. The amino acid carnitine may be involved and a daily dose of 1,000 mg of bioflavonoids with 1,000 mg of vitamin C have also been beneficial.

## THREONINE

**Source:** Threonine is readily available from most protein foods including fish, chicken, beef, soybeans, liver, eggs, beans and milk. Corn and rice are fairly low in threonine.

**Function:** Threonine, along with many other amino acids, is an important constituent of collagen, elastin and enamel protein. When choline, a lipotropic substance, is deficient in the diet, threonine takes on the role of a lipotropic to prevent fatty buildup in the liver.

# HISTIDINE

**Source:** Histidine is readily available from most protein foods.

**Function:** Histidine is necessary for growth in children and probably is essential for adults since we can't manufacture it. But it is not classified as an essential amino acid for adults.

Histidine is the amino acid from which the biochemical substance histamine is derived. Both histidine and histamine can chelate or grab onto trace elements such as copper and zinc. In certain forms of arthritis there is a tissue overload of copper or other heavy metals. Because of the chelating properties of histidine, it is sometimes used in the treatment of arthritis to remove these heavy metals.

# REFERENCES

1. Kugler, H.J. 1973. *Slowing Down the Aging Process.* New York: Jove Publications. pp. 71, 148, 173.

2. Kugler, H.J. *American Laboratory.* 8, 24, Nov. 1976.

3. Cutting, W.C. 1972. *Handbook of Pharmacology.* New York: Appleton-Century Crofts. 5th ed: pp. 251-252.

4. Crawford, M.D. *Lancet* 1, p. 942. 1962.

5. Foy, J.M., and Parratt, J.R. *Lancet* 1, p. 942. 1962.

6. Aylward, M. *IRCS Med. Sci.* 1: 30, 1973.

7. Stein, G.; Milton, F.; Bebbington, P.; Wood, K.; Coppen, A. *Br. Med. J.* 11: 547, 1976.

8. Zuckerman, M. and Lubin, B. 1965. Educational and industrial testing service. San Diego, CA.

9. Hildreth, H.M. *J. Clin. Psychol.* 2: 214, 1946.

10. Bridges, P.K.; Bartlett, J.R.; Sepping, P.; Kantamaneni, B.D.; Curzon, V. *Psychol. Med.* 6: 399, 1976.

11. Jensen, K.; Fruensgaard, K.; Ahlfors, U.G.; Pinkanen, T.A.; Tuomikoski, S.; Ose, E.; Dencker, S.J.; Lindberg, D.; Nagy, A. *Lancet* II: 920, 1975.

12. Broadhurst, A.D. and Arenillas, L. *Curr. Med. Res. Opinion* 3: 413, 1975.

13. Chouinard, G.; Young, G.N.; Annable, L.; Sourkes, T.L. *Br. Med. J.* I: 1422, 1978.

14. Herrington, R.N.; Bruce, A.; Johnstone, E.C.; Lader, M.H. *Psychol. Med.* 6: 673, 1976.

15. Cooper, A.J. *Psychopharmacology* 61: 97-102, 1979.

16. Brainard, John B. 1977. *Control of Migraine.* New York: Norton.

17. Sicuteri, Federigo. *Headache* vol. 13, pp. 19-22, April 1973.

18. Anthony, Michael. *Research in Clinical Studies in Headache.* vol. 6, pp. 110-116, 1978.

19. Dreizen, Samuel. *International J. of Vitamin and Nutrition Research* vol. 49, p. 220, 1979.

20. Shive, William. *Biochemical and Nutritional Aspects of Alcoholism.* Symposium, Austin: University of Texas, pp. 17-25, 1965.

21. Cottlier, E. *J.A.M.A.* vol. 244, no. 23, pp. 2593-4, Dec. 12, 1980.

22. Eustace, Barton-Wright. *Medical World News.* October 7, 1978.

23. Finkelstein, Cello and Kyle. *Biochem. Biophys. Res. Commum.* 61: 525, 1974.

24. Khaleeluddin, K. and Philpott, W. Data Sheet, Philpott Medical Center, Oklahoma City, OK, 1980.

25. Gelenberg, A. *Am. J. Psychiatry* 137: 622-23, 1980.

26. Tankersley, R.W. Amino acid requirements of herpes simplex virus in human cells. *J. Bact.* 87: 609-613, 1964.

27. Kagan, C. Lysine therapy for herpes simplex. *Lancet* 1: 127, Jan. 26, 1974.

28. Griffith, R.S., Norins, A.L. and Kagan, C. A multicentered study of lysine therapy in herpes simplex infection. *Dermatologica* 156: 257-267, 1978.